charting

THE SYSTEMATIC APPROACH TO ACHIEVING CONTROL

by Janice L. Roth,
R.N., B.S.N., C.D.E.

Diabetes Self-Management Books
New York

CHARTING: The Systematic Approach to Achieving Control.

 This book was originally published as a series of articles in *Diabetes Self-Management*, a bimonthly publication of R.A. Rapaport Publishing, Inc., 150 West 22nd Street, New York, NY 10011.

 Diabetes Self-Management thanks the Diabetes Control foundation for giving them permission to reproduce their charts and portions thereof and for allowing *Diabetes Self-Management* to draw heavily on their instructional material.

Additional copies may be ordered directly from the publisher. Write to *Diabetes Self-Management Books*, 150 West 22nd Street, New York, NY 10011.

Director of Special Projects: James Hazlett
Director of Manufacturing: Maryanne Schott
Project Editor: Beverly Logan
Art Director: Richard Boland
Printed in the United States of America

ISBN 0-9631701-0-4

First Printing 1990
Second Printing 1991

INTRODUCTION

Perhaps the most important reason to achieve good control is to feel good every day, and to have the energy you need for living your life the way you want to live it. If your blood glucose levels have been high, you can bet that much of the glucose from the foods you're eating is staying in your blood rather than getting into the body tissues where it is needed. This may be because your body is producing too little insulin or because your body tissues are not responding well to the insulin that is present. The result is usually fatigue. Achieving good control can give you a dramatic increase in energy levels and, with that, a renewed sense of well-being and a positive emotional outlook. Good diabetes control can also prevent those unwanted highs and lows that can sometimes turn into an emergency (such as insulin shock or diabetic ketoacidosis), as well as long-term complications of the diabetes.

This book can help you achieve and maintain good control by showing you how to keep systematic records and how to apply the results in a simple, straightforward way. Please notice that this book has no table of contents. This is not an accident; the only way to achieve an understanding of the system described in this book is to start out at the beginning and read through to the end—in other words, to build your knowledge step by step. Part One describes the step-by-step approach to analyzing your body's daily response to your diabetes program. Part Two offers solutions to common problems. And Part Three provides a checklist for tackling control problems.

Remember that this book is not intended to replace your health-care professional. Rather, our aim is to give you a powerful tool that will enhance the ability of you and your doctor, working together, to make decisions regarding your management.

PART ONE
GETTING STARTED

Step 1
Food First

Whether you have Type I (insulin-dependent) diabetes or Type II (non-insulin-dependent) diabetes, the first step must be to establish a healthy meal plan. It must be appropriate in terms of total daily calories and distribution of carbohydrate, fat, and protein, and must be consistent from day to day.

Many people try to reduce high blood sugars merely by increasing doses of insulin or diabetes pills. If you try this before establishing a basic meal plan, good control will not only be difficult to achieve, but you may experience side effects such as unwanted weight gain. This happens because calories which "spilled" into the urine when blood glucose was too high become stored as fat when medication is increased and blood sugars become more normal. You can avoid this by setting the right calorie level for gradual weight loss and then adjusting the medication to achieve normal blood sugars.

Those who take insulin will often have erratic blood sugars when their meal plan is inappropriate or inconsistent. For instance, if 8 units of Regular insulin works well to help you use today's 400-calorie breakfast, it will be too much tomorrow morning if you eat only 200 calories for breakfast—and low blood sugar will result. Guessing how much insulin you need for a particular meal and changing your dose every day can be a dangerous game that seldom results in normal blood sugars. It is much better to plan to eat consistent amounts every day and to adjust your insulin based on the patterns or trends that become apparent as you do regular blood glucose testing.

How do you get started on the road to good control with the right meal plan? Your physician or dietitian can calculate how many calories your body needs by considering your height, weight, age, body frame type, and activity level. To lose weight gradually, eat about 500 calories per day less than what your body needs (to gain weight, eat 500 calories per day more than you would need). For instance, if your body needs 2000 calories per day to maintain body functions but you eat only 1500 calories, then 500 calories each day will be pulled from your body's fat stores. If you follow this meal plan for 7 days, you should use 7 x 500 calories of body fat (3500 calories) and you will lose one pound. A steady pound-per-week loss may get you to your goal weight faster and healthier than the crash diets you may have tried in the past.

Many times it is difficult to follow a preprinted diet sheet either because no one explains the concept of "points" or "exchanges," or because the diet doesn't fit your particular needs for meal timing or food preferences. If this is the case, then you would benefit from having a meal plan designed to accommodate your specific needs and food preferences. Your doctor or local diabetes association can help you find a registered dietitian (RD) or certified diabetes educator (CDE) who can develop such a plan for you, give you the training you need to comfortably follow the meal plan every day, and show you how to adjust to unusual circumstances such as traveling, eating out, or sick days. Many cities now have comprehensive diabetes education programs that provide excellent instruction in the use of a meal plan.

Step 2
Blood Glucose Monitoring

The next step toward good control is performing frequent, regular glucose monitoring to see how your meal plan and medication are working to keep your blood sugar within a normal range. Blood glucose self-monitoring is rapidly replacing urine testing because it is far more accurate, as well as easy and affordable. Doing your own blood sugar tests helps you to see patterns of low or high blood sugars at different times of the day, and it gives you and your doctor information on which to base changes in your diabetes medication. This is far better than guesswork or performing just one blood sugar test in the lab or doctor's office every few weeks or months. If you have unusual symptoms from time to time, a quick blood test can help to determine if the symptoms are due to abnormal blood sugar levels. Blood glucose testing also helps you see when small adjustments need to be made in your food or medication in response to exercise, illness, or stress.

The minimum supplies needed to start blood glucose testing include a container of visual strips, such as Chemstrip bG, and a spring-loaded device with small disposable lancets that puncture your finger virtually painlessly. Blood glucose meters now come in a variety of sizes and shapes and are moderately priced. Many insurance companies will cover at least 80% of the cost of a meter, especially if you are using insulin.

Whether you decide to test your blood by matching the visual strip to a color chart or by using a blood glucose meter, you'll want to get started right away. You'll be amazed at how much easier it is to control your diabetes when you know what's really going on within your body. However, be sure you get the training you need to perform your tests accurately; your pharmacist or a supplier may be able to train you in their use. If not, be sure you seek help from another reliable source, such as your diabetes association, your physician's office, or your diabetes educator. It is a waste of your time and money and could even be dangerous if you base your medication changes on inaccurate results. Recording your test results in a record book or chart will help you and your doctor get a clear picture of your blood glucose patterns.

Step 3
Exercise

Regular exercise is the next important step in your diabetes management routine. Following a regular exercise program can have many benefits: increased sensitivity of your body tissues to insulin, decreased blood sugar levels, improved cardiovascular fitness, better muscle tone and flexibility, and prevention of calcium loss from the bone. In addition, most people who exercise regularly feel better about themselves and have a better attitude toward life in general.

Before you get started, discuss with your doctor the types of exercise you are interested in to find out if there are any physical reasons why you shouldn't try a particular type. Your doctor also may want to monitor your heart more closely—especially if you have had heart problems in the past, if you are over 40, or if heart problems tend to run in your family.

Aerobic exercise does your body the most good. Common aerobic choices include brisk walking, bicycling, and swimming. You may need some help in choosing the best exercise routine for you, as well as some instruction in the basics, such as figuring out your target heart rate, stretching at the start of each exercise session, and ways to warm up and cool down before and after your exercise session.

Your local YMCA counselor may be able to help, or your doctor may suggest a session with a registered physical therapist at a hospital or physical medicine clinic. Be sure you get the help you need so that your exercise session is designed to do your body the most good and so that you minimize the possibility of an exercise-related injury.

As you begin to exercise regularly, you will want to monitor your blood glucose levels closely and work with a doctor or nurse educator to adjust your food or medicine to accommodate the increase in activity. For instance, before you engage in a strenuous physical activity such as an hour of tennis, you should achieve a balance by either having an extra snack before or during the exercise or by decreasing the dose of insulin that will be acting at that particular time of day. Keeping a close record of your amounts and typos of physical activity and your blood sugar response to them will give you useful information when making adjustments.

Step 4
Charting

Charting is the vital part of your diabetes management program that ties it all together and helps you make progress toward better control. To consistently achieve normal blood sugar levels requires some careful investigation of all the components of your management program so you can see where you achieved good results or where you might change an aspect of your program for better control. Details about portions eaten, blood glucose test results, times and amounts of insulin taken, and low blood sugar reactions are far too numerous to rely on your memory alone. You will want to be able to analyze your results daily, weekly, or monthly to determine developing trends and make appropriate changes. You and your doctor will appreciate your careful record-keeping when you discuss any necessary changes in your program. In addition, careful recording makes you more accountable to yourself for the success of your self-care program. For instance, several elevated morning sugar tests in a week's time might be easily forgotten if not written down. But if you see them all on paper at the end of the week, you can see if there is a problem requiring your attention. You might be able to recognize that the larger-than-usual bedtime snack is the culprit behind each elevated morning test.

Take a look at the sample chart on pages 8 and 9, which we'll explain a step at a time. First, the top of the chart is filled out with the name, the day of the week and date, and the weight in pounds or kilograms. (To convert kilograms to pounds, multiply the number of kilograms by 2.2.)

Blood glucose tests. The center third of the daily chart is a graph for displaying the results of your blood glucose tests. The unit of measurement we use in the United States to express blood glucose is milligrams of glucose per deciliter of blood (mg/dl). The range between 50 and 150 mg/dl is shaded on the chart to indicate what might be considered an acceptable blood glucose range. (A person who does not have diabetes would have sugar levels ranging from 70 to 130 mg/dl.) For a person who has diabetes and requires insulin to control it, the shaded area represents significant control. If you are a senior citizen or don't feel any early warning symptoms of low blood sugar reactions, your doctor may define a slightly different goal for your acceptable blood glucose range—for instance, 80–170 mg/dl. The fasting blood sugar (taken before you eat anything in the morning) is usually one of the lowest readings of the day. For tight control this should not exceed 120 mg/dl, and for fairly good control it should not exceed 140 mg/dl. Be sure to talk with your doctor about a glucose range you can agree on.

You will be testing and recording changes in your blood glucose levels to understand what causes those changes. The blood test results should be written in the appropriate spaces just above the top of the graph section. These are the seven times each day that are most often recommended for testing. There is also a space for recording the time of an additional test and its results. In the sample chart, Joe's test before breakfast on August 20 was 79 mg/dl.

The next step is to graph the results. The top and the bottom lines of the graph section are time lines. They run from midnight to midnight, with noon (N) in the middle. Each hour is divided into four quarters of 15 minutes each. The scales at the left and right sides of the graph section show blood glucose levels in mg/dl. On the chart these range from 0 at the bottom to 400 at the top. Enter the blood test result to the nearest 10 mg/dl, and to the nearest quarter hour. The sample chart shows a recorded blood glucose of 79 mg/dl at 6 AM before breakfast. In preparing your own graph, you would enter each test result in the appropriate spaces above the graph, and then record the result in the graph with a bold dot. When you finish recording and graphing all the tests for the day, draw a line to connect each consecutive dot. This gives you your blood glucose profile for the day. Notice that the points on your profile will correspond to the written record of test results. Before long, you will begin to see patterns in these profiles from day to day, and by understanding them, you can learn to manage your diabetes better. Since Joe tested seven times on August 20, we have a very clear picture of his blood glucose fluctuations through the day. You may not need to test seven times, but you should test at least four times daily if you are using insulin and are striving for better control.

Insulin. On your chart, you should select and circle the letter that stands for the type or types of insulin you use:

- N/L for NPH or Lente (intermediate-acting insulins)
- R/S for Regular or Semilente (short-acting insulins)
- P/U for Protamine Zinc or Ultra-Lente (long-acting insulins)

If you are using a premixed insulin such as 70/30 or Mixtard, write this in next to N/L and circle it. Next, indicate with an arrowhead (^) under the lower time line the time (to the nearest quarter-hour) when you injected your insulin. Write under the arrowhead the number of units of each kind of insulin that you injected. In the example on the sample chart, Joe took 18 units of NPH and 9 units of Regular at 6 AM. He took 9 units of Regular at 6 PM (before supper); the " + 3" indicates that he took 3 units more than his usual before-supper dose of 6 units of Regular. At 11 PM (his bedtime), he took 7 units of NPH.

Insulin sites. Record the site where you gave your insulin on the "Site" line under the number of units given. You may want to develop a system for numbering the specific injection site within a given area. For instance, you might be able to give insulin in 12 different sites on one arm, and they could be identified according to a chart such as the one in Figure 1. On the chart you could identify the site used by listing the part of the body and then the specific site number next to it. In the sample chart, Joe gave his morning insulin on site number 6 of his abdomen.

FIGURE 1.
Sample of Injection Rotation Diagram.

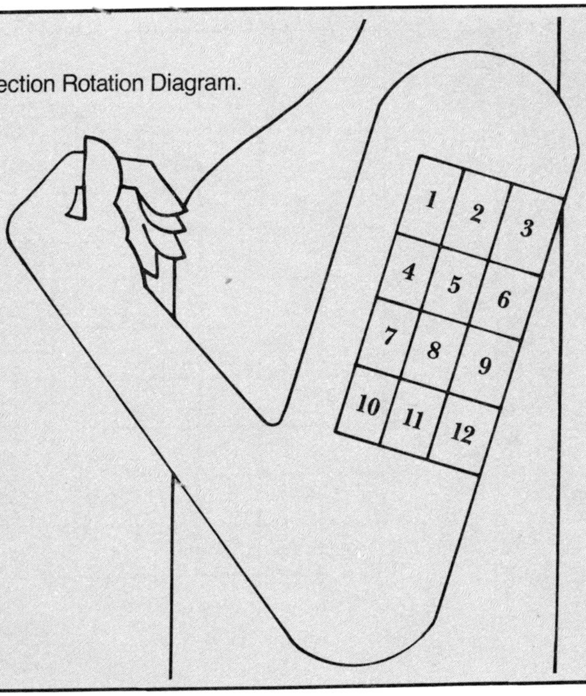

Name JOE MACALUSO **Day** TUESDAY **Date** AUG. 20

Weight: 167 Lbs: Kg: Analysis: LAID UP 60-POUND BLOCKS IN A.M. LOT OF PRESSURE. SITE SHUT DOWN IN P.M. DUE TO RAIN. LIGHT CARPENTRY AT HOME. TOOK 3 EXTRA UNITS OF REGULAR BEFORE DINNER FOR ICE CREAM.

Before Break.	After Break.	Before Lunch	After Lunch	Before Supper	After Supper	Bed Time	Other	Time
79	112	46	75	101	127	83		

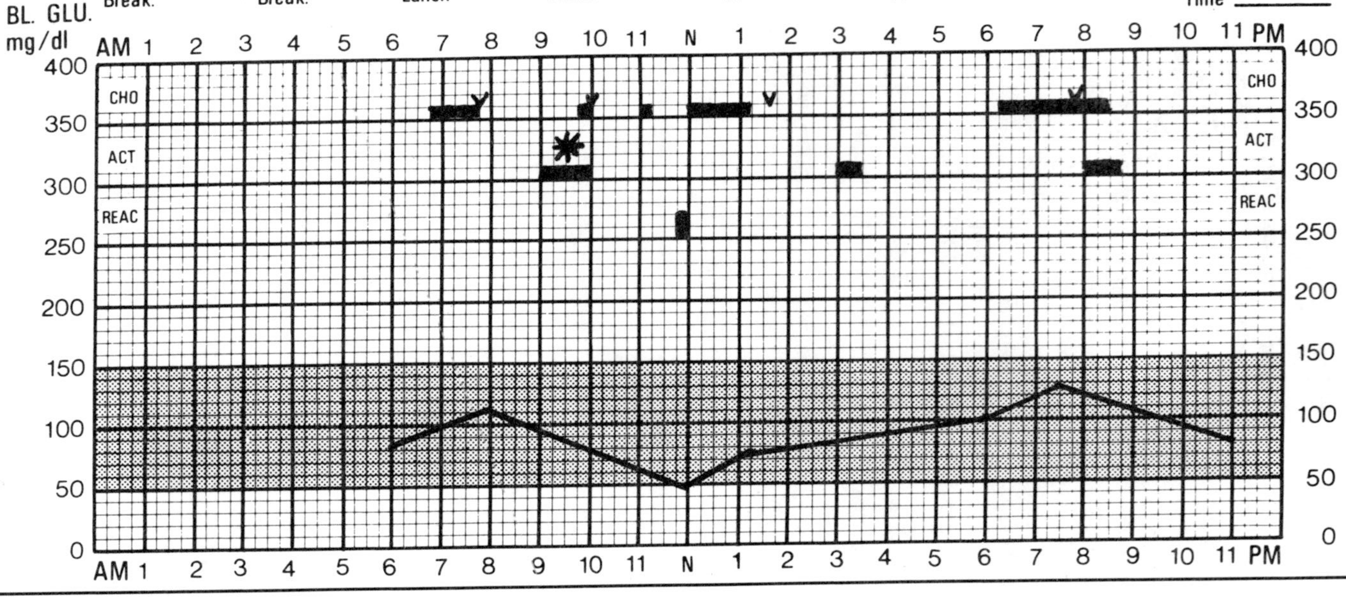

Time	AM 1	2	3	4	5	6	7	8	9	10	11	N	1	2	3	4	5	6	7	8	9	10	11 PM
Ins.						^												^					^
(N)/L						18																	7
(R)/S						9												9 (+3)					
P/U																							
Site						ABDOMEN 6												L. ARM 3					L. THIGH 9

BREAKFAST - SNACKS	Quota: 40:10		LUNCH - SNACKS	Quota: 65		SUPPER - SNACKS	Quota: 65	
Time: 6:45	MEA-SURE	GMS CHO	Time: 12:00	MEA-SURE	GMS CHO	Time: 6:15	MEA-SURE	GMS CHO
BOILED EGGS	2	1	MEAT SAND.	2	48	LAMB CHOPS	2	—
BACON	1	—	RAW CARROTS	1	4	HASH BROWNS	1/2 C.	26
HI-FIBER TOAST	1	12	SMALL APPLE	1/2	5	SPINACH, CR.	1 C.	5
WHEATIES	1 C.	23	COFFEE	2	—	SQUASH	1/2 C.	12
MILK	1/2 C.	6				DIET WAFERS	3	9
					57	ICE CREAM	1/2 C.	(26)
		42				MILK	1 C.	12
9:45								
GRAPEFRUIT JUICE	1/2 C.	9						90
11:00								
MILK	3/4 C.	(9)						

Food. Your dietitian may have suggested a quota of calories, exchanges, or grams of carbohydrates (CHO) for each meal. If you are using grams of CHO to calculate your diet, record your quota in the space next to "Quota" on the food chart on the bottom third of the page.

Write the time you start each meal in the "Time" spaces. Write what you ate or drank at each meal or snack in the appropriate column. Write the total quantity beside each food in the "Measure" column. If you are counting grams of CHO, record them in the adjoining column. If you are using an exchange system in your diet, you could write the exchanges in the "Measure" column instead of recording the specific quantity. Feel free to individualize this section of the chart so that it will help keep track of your intake with whichever system or systems you are using.

The total number of grams of CHO in any meal or snack is transferred in block form to the top line of the chart's graph section, labeled "CHO." Start your CHO

FIGURE 2.
Example of a Daily Activity Scale.

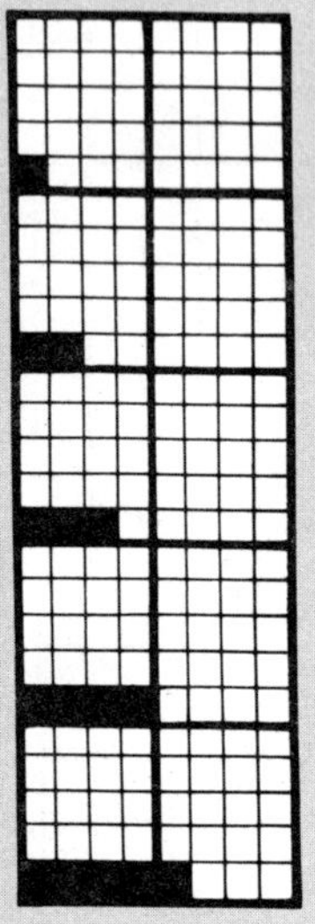

1 means minimal activity.

2 means less than usual activity.

3 means average activity.

4 means more than usual activity.

5 means maximal activity.

FIGURE 3.
Grading Reactions.

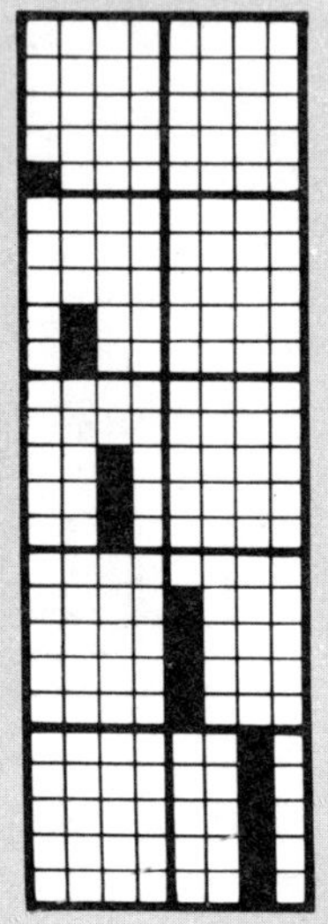

1 means you don't feel "quite right." You may ask, "Am I having a reaction or not?"

2 means your usual symptoms of a reaction.

3 means your symptoms are intensified. You may feel panic.

4 means you may be confused and/or argumentative. You may not realize you're having a reaction. You may require assistance.

5 means you lost consciousness.

block at the line which represents (to the nearest quarter-hour) when you began to eat, and fill in one small square for each 10 grams of CHO. Use an arrowhead to indicate your CHO quota for each meal or snack, so you can compare the amount of CHO you actually ate with the amount in your quota. This will help you consider the predictable effect changes in your diet have on your blood glucose and will make the timing of your meals and snacks throughout the day clear to you and to your health-care team. It will also illustrate the kinds of adjustments you may need to make in insulin or activity when you eat meals with varying carbohydrate concentrations. A small book listing the CHO content of foods is available in most book stores if you don't have one.

Grading activity. Your insulin and your diet have been calculated for everyday needs, but your daily activities may vary significantly from day to day. Think about the day you are charting in terms of how your activity has been different from your usual activity. Use a scale of 1 to 5 such as the one in Figure 2 to grade your day's activity as it compares with *your own normal activity*. The lower the number, the less activity it represents. As you can see, a grade of 3 represents average activity for a particular period.

Activity is charted on the second line of the graph section, which is labeled "ACT." Record activity for the morning in the area between your breakfast and your lunch, your afternoon's activity between lunch and supper, and the evening's activity between supper and bedtime. On the sample chart, we can see that Joe's morning rating of 4 means he was more active than he usually is in the morning, and his afternoon rating of 2 means he was less active than usual. His activity in the evening was graded 3, or equal to his typical amount of activity for the evening.

Insulin reactions. Insulin reactions, like activity, are graded on a scale of 1 to 5 with 1 being the least serious and 5 the most serious. Insulin reactions are charted vertically to make them stand out on the chart. Figure 3 shows the different grades of severity. You may not have experienced all five grades of a reaction.

Stress. Even everyday kinds of stress can cause swings in your blood glucose. If you record when you are feeling stressed, it can help you learn the effect of stress on your blood glucose control. Use an asterisk (*) in the activity space (ACT) to show the times you felt stressed. In the sample chart, Joe has recorded that he felt stressed during mid-morning.

Step 5
Analysis and Response

Each completed chart contains detailed information about the effect of separate variables upon your blood glucose. About once a week, arrange your charts in sequence on a flat surface to identify repeating patterns of change in blood glucose levels. With practice, you can learn to predict your blood glucose responce to various repeated actions, such as changes in your diet or level of activity. You will

Name JOE MACALUSO Insulin Types: N / R Period Starting 4 / 20 Ending 5 / 17

Date	Day	Blood Glucose Tests							Insulins				Reac.	Comments
		Breakfast		Lunch		Supper		Bed Time	Before				AM	
		Before	After	Before	After	Before	After		Break.	Lunch	Supper	Bed	PM	
4/20	Mon.	119	146			74	113		18 / 9		6	7		
4/21	Tues.			58	130			121						
4/22	Wed.	83		51		79								
4/23	Thu.		138	47			(162)	(195)					11:15	SOMOGYI?
4/24	Fri.	72		63		82		113						
4/25	Sat.	101	149		148	112		131						
4/26	Sun.			107				116						SLEPT LATE
4/27	Mon.	86		52		138								
4/28	Tues.	140					(174)	(211)						SORE THROAT
4/29	Wed.	(236)		(227)		(290)			20 / 11		7	9		FEVER
4/30	Thu.	(183)		(175)		(168)			19 / 10		6	8		"
5/1	Fri.			86			142		18 / 9			7		
5/2	Sat.	—	—	—	—	—	—							TRAVELLING

5/3	Sun.		127	46	133			148					11:30	SPLITTING WOOD
5/4	Mon.	124		48		137							11:45	
5/5	Tues.		139		143		126							
5/6	Wed.	117	144	51	139	82	146	112				9		Italian Dinner
5/7	Thu.			69		106		134	8			6		Too many AM Reac
5/8	Fri.	98		81			137							
5/9	Sat.		141											
5/10	Sun.				(193)	(208)	(152)					8		Mother's Day
5/11	Mon.					87		98				6		
5/12	Tues.	148		76		127								
5/13	Wed.		136		142		(152)							
5/14	Thu.	121		63		138								
5/15	Fri.		143					149						
5/16	Sat.	98		51		101							12:15	PICNIC LUNCH
5/17	Sun.	119	150	97		72	141							

<55 >(150)

want to work with your diabetes-care professional to consider what adjustments might need to be made in amounts or timing of your meals, snacks, medication, or activity levels to prevent unwanted swings in blood glucose outside the normal range. As you finish a day's chart, think about the events you have recorded that influenced your control. Make a note in the "Analysis" section at the top of the chart about what you think the chart shows. Try to include some strategy for how you could handle the same or similar experiences better another time.

Monthly chart. While the daily chart is most useful for gaining understanding of individual variables and for achieving initial control, the simpler monthly chart (pages 12–13) will often be enough for maintaining records of good control. When you have learned the effect of individual variables and have achieved some measure of improved control, you may prefer to move to the less detailed (and less demanding) monthly charts. From time to time, however, you may decide to return briefly to full daily charting to solve a particular management problem.

Some people who have Type II diabetes and use diabetes pills or diet alone to control their diabetes may be testing less often than those on insulin. They may prefer the less complicated monthly chart for their regular recording.

The monthly chart contains four weeks of data divided into four one-week sections. You will be recording the date, blood glucose levels measured before or after meals, amounts of insulin taken, and insulin reactions. The "Comments" section can be used to record any details of the day that were significant in terms of your control.

In the "Insulins" column, the usual dose is recorded at the top. To keep the chart uncluttered you may want to record only the changes in the amount underneath. If you are using a diabetes pill, you could write the name and amount taken in the "Insulins" column.

To analyze the monthly chart, first decide on an acceptable range for your blood glucose levels. (The daily charts use a range of 50–150 mg/dl, but that may not be appropriate for your individual needs.) Then mark all test results that fall *outside* that range. We have underlined low results, and circled high results. Try to identify patterns so you can plan an appropriate response in terms of your diet, medication, and activity, or a plan of action to prevent them in the future. If you are testing less frequently, establish a random pattern of tests that will yield some information each week about each of the testing periods.

If you have difficulty interpreting results on the monthly chart, try changing back to the daily sheets for a week or two. Once the glucose pattern is back to where you want it, you can return to the monthly chart.

Initially, these charting projects may seem to be a lot of paper work, but they will be worth the trouble when you begin to see and understand your body's reactions to your self-management program. This understanding and your response will help put *you* in control of your diabetes, rather than letting it control you. Even if you've always thought of yourself as "brittle," there's hope for more stable control through the use of this or a similar system. It will allow you to become a partner with your physician in making the decisions in your self-management program. You are the one most familiar with your body, and you'll have written proof of it. The time and effort spent testing, recording, and analyzing will pay important dividends in your sense of control over your own life.

PART TWO
SOLVING COMMON PROBLEMS

So far, we have outlined a comprehensive system of daily and monthly charting for keeping track of your diabetes self-management routine, including dosages, meals and snacks, injection sites, activity, stress, and low blood sugar reactions. Now, we'll show you how to use the system to solve several common management problems. The sample charts that follow represent information collected over a number of days that reveal particular patterns that warrant attention. In the suggested solutions, you will notice that insulin adjustment is only one part of the program that can be altered to improve control. Content and timing of meals and snacks, timing and duration of activity, injection-site rotation, insulin types and their peaks, and stress management are some of the other aspects that may also be considered and adjusted.

In reviewing the sample cases, you may recognize a problem pattern similar to one that you have had in the past or are currently experiencing. It is important to remember that the solution in your particular case should be handled by you and your health-care professional; the suggested solutions may not work for everyone. However, the cases should give you "food for thought" regarding different aspects of your diabetes self-management program that could be adjusted to improve control.

Remember, the sample charts we will discuss do not represent monitoring results from a single day of testing but rather the patterns which result after a number of days. When analyzing *your* data, don't spend a great deal of time trying to explain a single blood glucose result, but rather look for the trends or patterns that develop over time.

Daytime Descending

With this pattern, the fasting (morning) blood glucose is elevated and control gradually improves during the day. Your first effort toward achieving control should be to "fix" the fasting level and then focus on the other blood sugars. In Figure 4 (page 17) the problem is the duration of the morning insulin injection. NPH, though intermediate in action, reaches its peak effect in 6 to 12 hours. By 18 hours its action is nearly finished. Thus, the injection taken at 7:00 AM is nearly exhausted by 1:00 AM. Because there is very little insulin in the system during the night, an elevated morning blood sugar is not surprising. In this case the blood sugar is most elevated in the morning, though it was likely climbing all night. This might be improved by adding a small dose of NPH at suppertime or bedtime and adjusting the dose as needed to get a normal fasting result.

Once you achieve normal fasting blood sugar, you may not require as much insulin during the day as you were used to. For instance, the dose required for normal blood sugar values over a 24-hour period for the person in Figure 4 might be 8 units Regular and 28 units NPH in the morning, and 12 units NPH at night. Most people will also require a small amount of fast-acting insulin (Regular or Semilente) before supper to achieve normal sugar during the evening hours.

A common question is, "Why do I need insulin during the night if I'm not eating?" The liver is capable of producing glucose by itself, particularly if it is not "guarded" by a steady baseline level of insulin during the night. This is especially true with persons who have Type II (non-insulin-dependent) diabetes requiring insulin. Another explanation for a rise in blood glucose in the early morning hours is called the "dawn phenomenon." This happens as the hormone systems in your body "wake up" several hours before you do. The hormones produced, especially cortisol and growth hormone, tend to have an opposite effect to insulin; thus the blood sugar rises. Your body requires insulin at all times to keep this trend in check. If you are striving for good blood sugar control, you will probably need at least two injections daily.

Rebound Effect

Another cause of high blood sugar in the morning is the rebound effect, which is also called the "Somogyi phenomenon" (shown in Figure 5, page 18). This is caused by too much longer-acting (Lente or NPH) insulin in the evening, which results in low blood sugar during the early morning hours (2:00 AM to 4:00 AM). Often this low blood sugar will not awaken you, but your body responds to it by producing hormones such as adrenaline, cortisol, and glucagon that raise your blood sugar. Sometimes these hormones cause the blood sugar to rebound to an abnormally high morning level. A decrease in the evening dose of Lente or NPH can prevent low blood sugar during the night, thus preventing this rebound effect.

Rather than change your insulin dose, this problem might be solved by increasing your bedtime snack, or by taking the suppertime dose of Lente or NPH at bedtime. Any time there is a pattern of high fasting blood sugars, test your blood sugar several days in a row at 3:00 AM to 4:00 AM (in addition to bedtime and fasting tests) to see what is happening during the night. Though the daytime blood sugar results are the same for the people in Figures 4 and 5, the night patterns are quite different, and the change in insulin dose needed is opposite. The person represented by Figure 4 needs to *increase* the evening insulin dose, and the person represented in Figure 5 needs to *decrease* the evening insulin dose.

Butterfly

The term "butterfly" means a similar blood sugar pattern in which both the morning and evening blood sugar values are elevated (see Figure 6, page 19). First, apply the rules for correcting fasting blood sugar, then focus on the remaining abnormal values. Once your fasting glucose is normal, the other blood sugars during the day often improve with the usual amount of daytime insulin.

The cause of high blood sugar levels in the evening hours is most often the result of an inadequate amount of insulin working during the evening. This can be remedied by taking additional Regular insulin before supper. The peak action of Regular insulin is two to four hours after the injection. Thus, Regular insulin taken before supper will "cover" the glucose in your supper. In Figure 6, you might begin by increasing the dose of presupper Regular to four or six units, continuing this dose for a few days. If your evening blood sugars are still elevated, you might

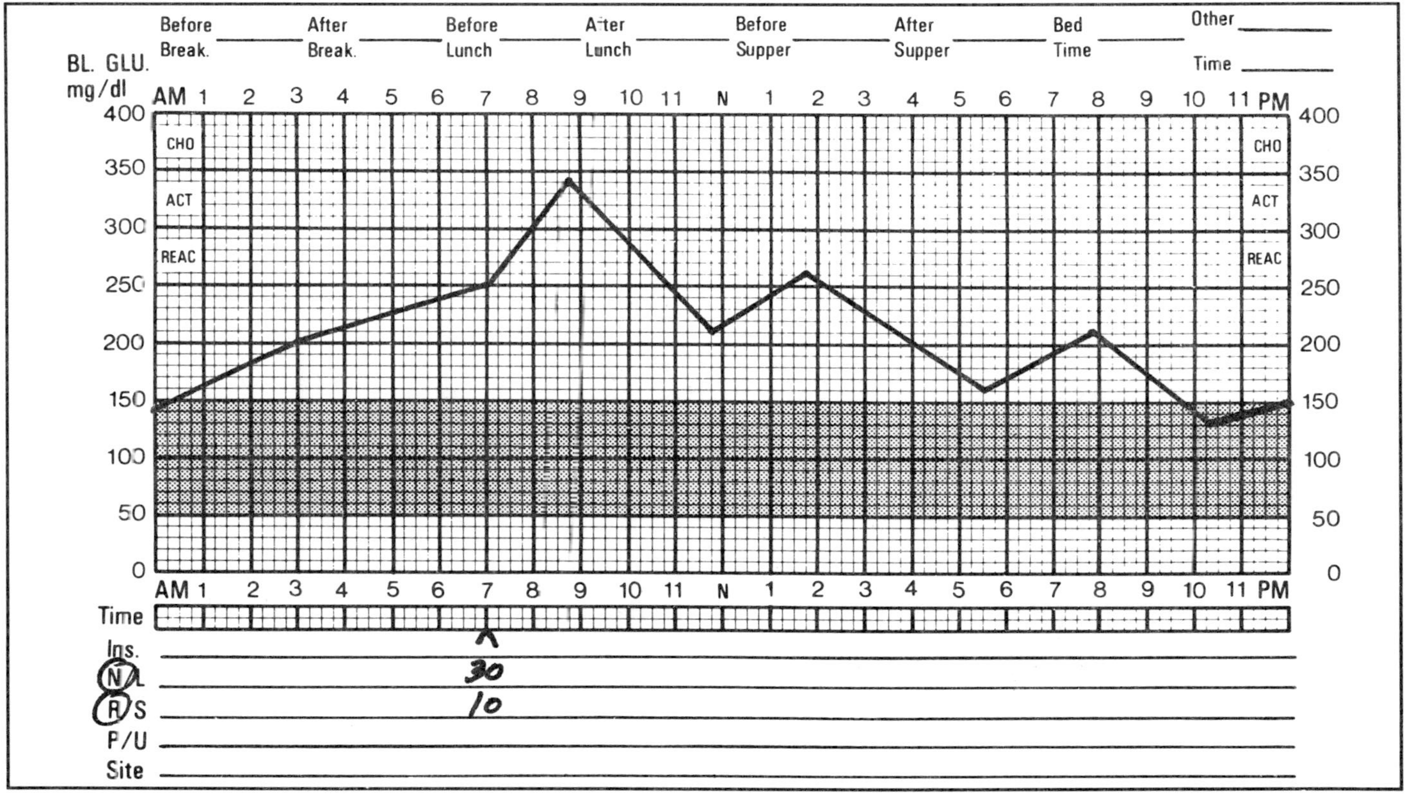

FIGURE 4. Example of *daytime descending*—fasting blood sugar is elevated; control improves during the day.

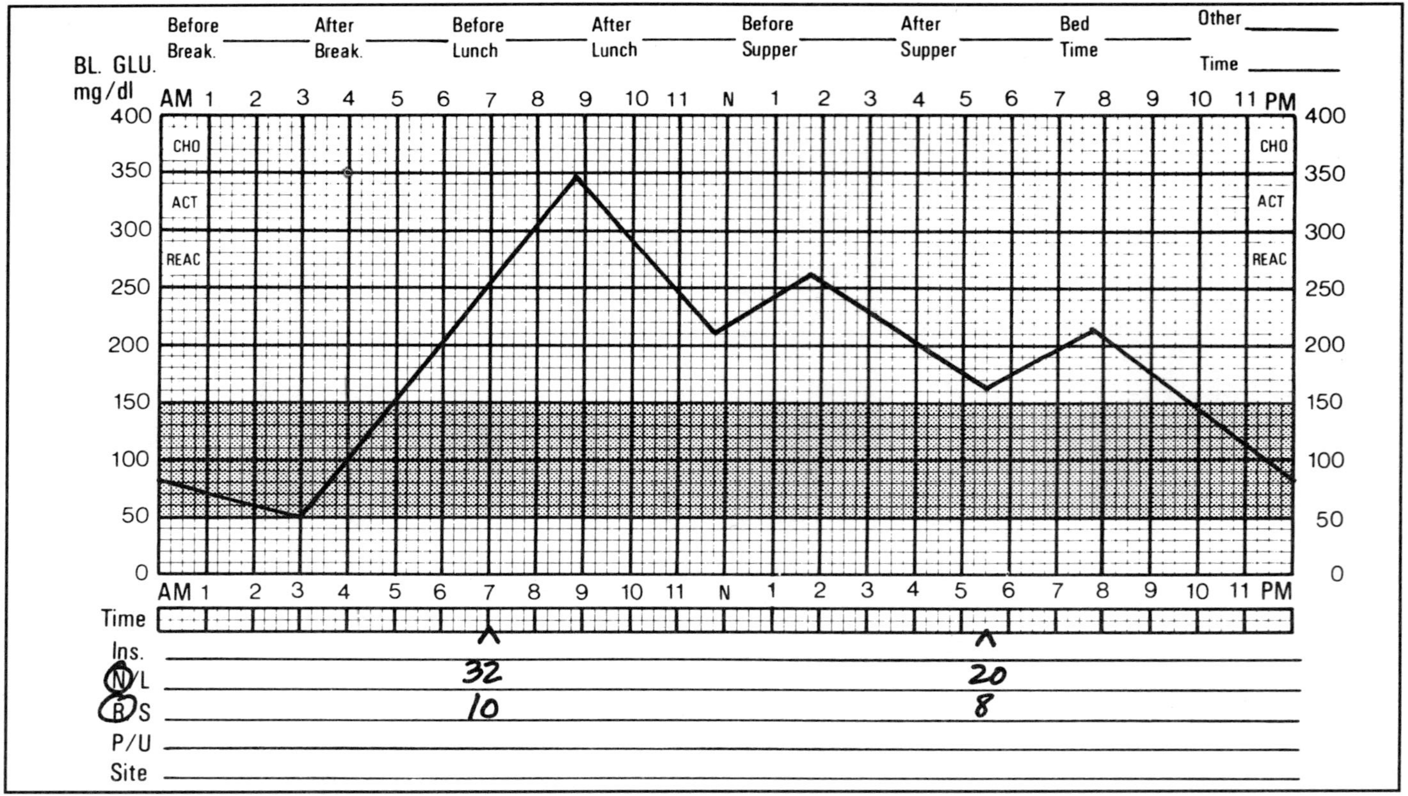

FIGURE 5. Example of the *rebound effect*—low blood sugar in the early morning hours.

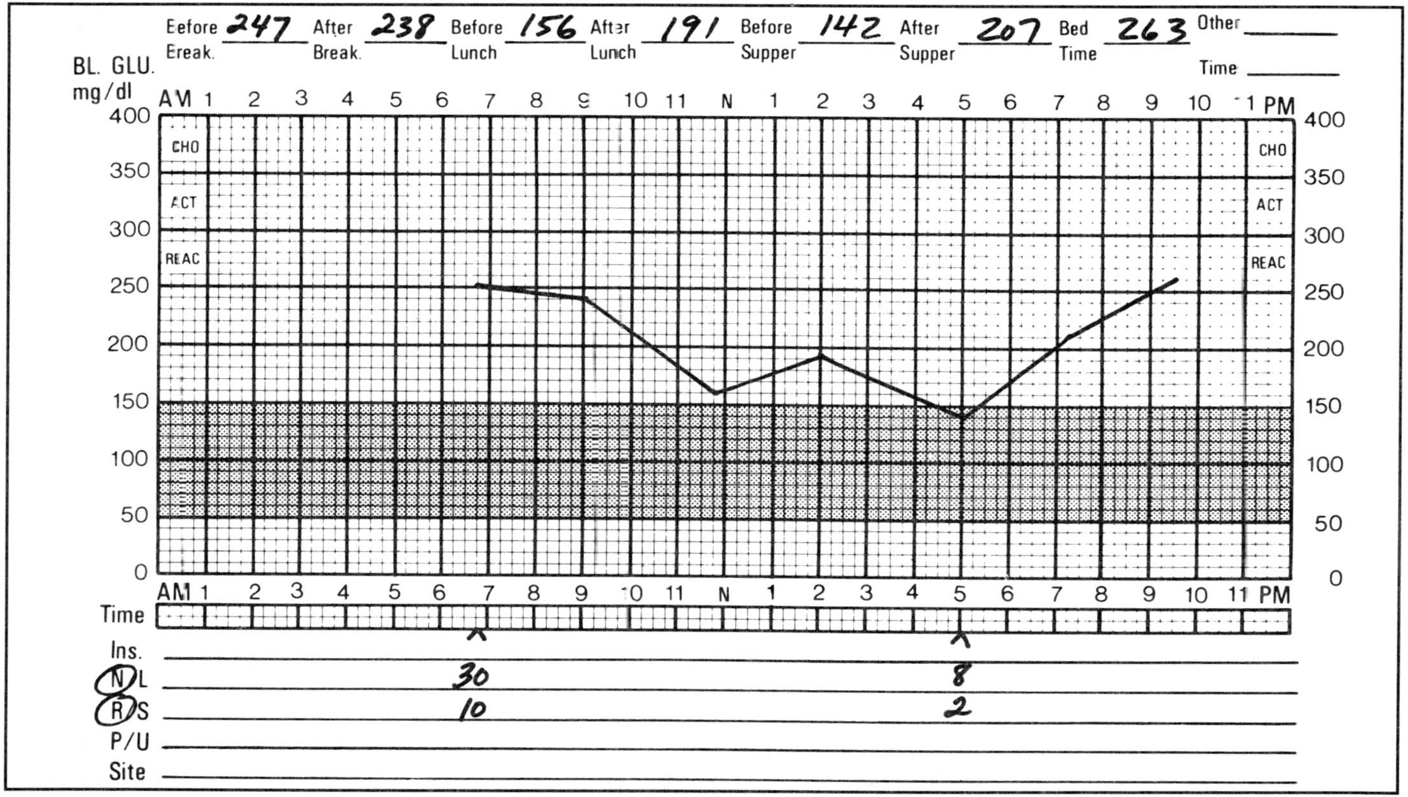

FIGURE 6. Example of the *butterfly*—both morning and evening blood sugars are elevated.

increase your evening dose of Regular by two units every two to three days until your evening sugar values are within normal range.

While making these changes, it is advisable to perform several tests at 3:00 AM to 4:00 AM to make sure your blood sugar is not falling too low during the night. After you have achieved normal evening blood sugars by raising the presupper dose of Regular, you may require slightly less NPH at supper to keep blood sugar levels normal during the night.

Another cause of elevated blood sugars during the evening is an overly large evening meal. In Part One we stressed the importance of first working with a diabetes-care professional to establish a balanced and appropriate meal plan before making major insulin adjustments. If you simply take more insulin to compensate for overly large meals, the result will be unwanted weight gain.

Overtreating Hypoglycemia

A third cause of high blood sugars in the evening is low blood sugar before supper (see Figure 7). This fellow's blood sugar was 283 mg/dl when tested at 9:00 PM. He could hardly believe the test, because he had low blood sugar before supper. When questioned further, he remembered that he had eaten a large candy bar to treat his hypoglycemia (insulin reaction) at 5:00 PM. The bedtime blood sugar had rebounded to 283 mg/dl as a result of the candy bar followed by his usual supper meal.

If there is a pattern of low blood sugar before dinner (occurring three or more times in one week), you should decrease the dose of NPH or Lente you take in the morning to prevent the low blood sugar before supper. This will prevent the "rebound" effect that results from the foods eaten to treat low blood sugar, or from your body's own hormonal response to hypoglycemia. An occasional low blood sugar before supper might be remedied by an increased afternoon snack, or by eating supper a little earlier. Whenever you have low blood sugar, respond appropriately with a reasonable amount of fast-acting carbohydrate, such as four ounces of orange juice or regular (non-diet) soda followed by a slower-acting carbohydrate and protein. If symptoms persist after 10 minutes, eat or drink a small, additional amount of a fast-acting sugar. Be careful though, because a large amount of carbohydrate, such as 12 ounces of soda or a large candy bar, will usually result in rebound hyperglycemia.

Testing your blood when you suspect hypoglycemia and continuing to test every 15 minutes until your blood sugar returns to normal will help you decide on the kinds and amounts of food you need to treat the low blood sugar appropriately to avoid rebounds.

Blood Sugar Peaks

One of the most common problems in diabetes control is a pattern of blood sugar elevation, or a peak, that occurs at one particular time of day. As shown in Figure 8 (page 22), rising blood sugar is recorded during the morning hours. Since a morning dose of Regular insulin peaks in the late morning, a simple increase in the dosage solved the problem.

By contrast, Figure 9 (page 23) shows elevated blood sugar in the late afternoon. This person was taking 30 units of 70/30 insulin in the morning (this type of insulin is 70% NPH and 30% Regular insulin prepared together in a stable mixture:

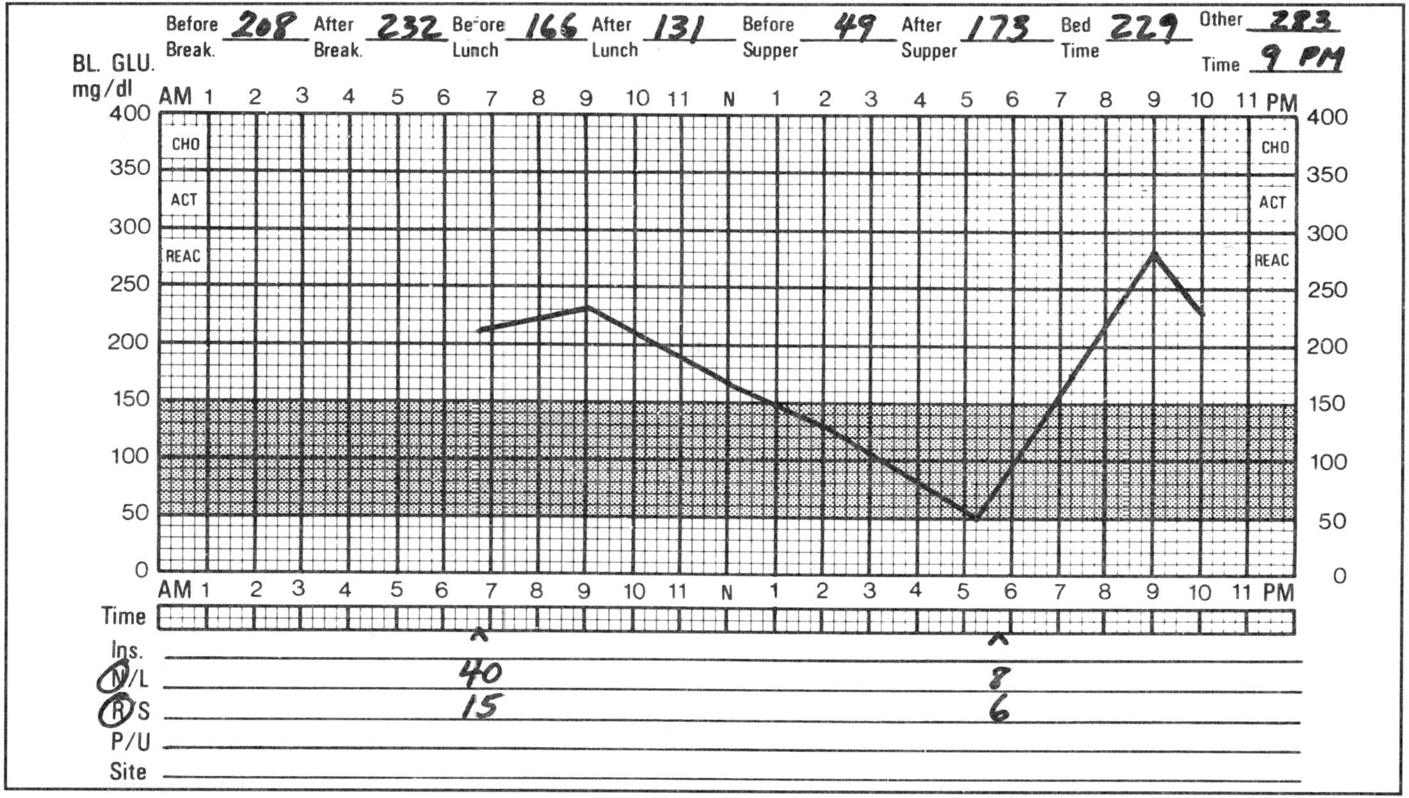

FIGURE 7. Example of hypoglycemia in the evening hours before supper.

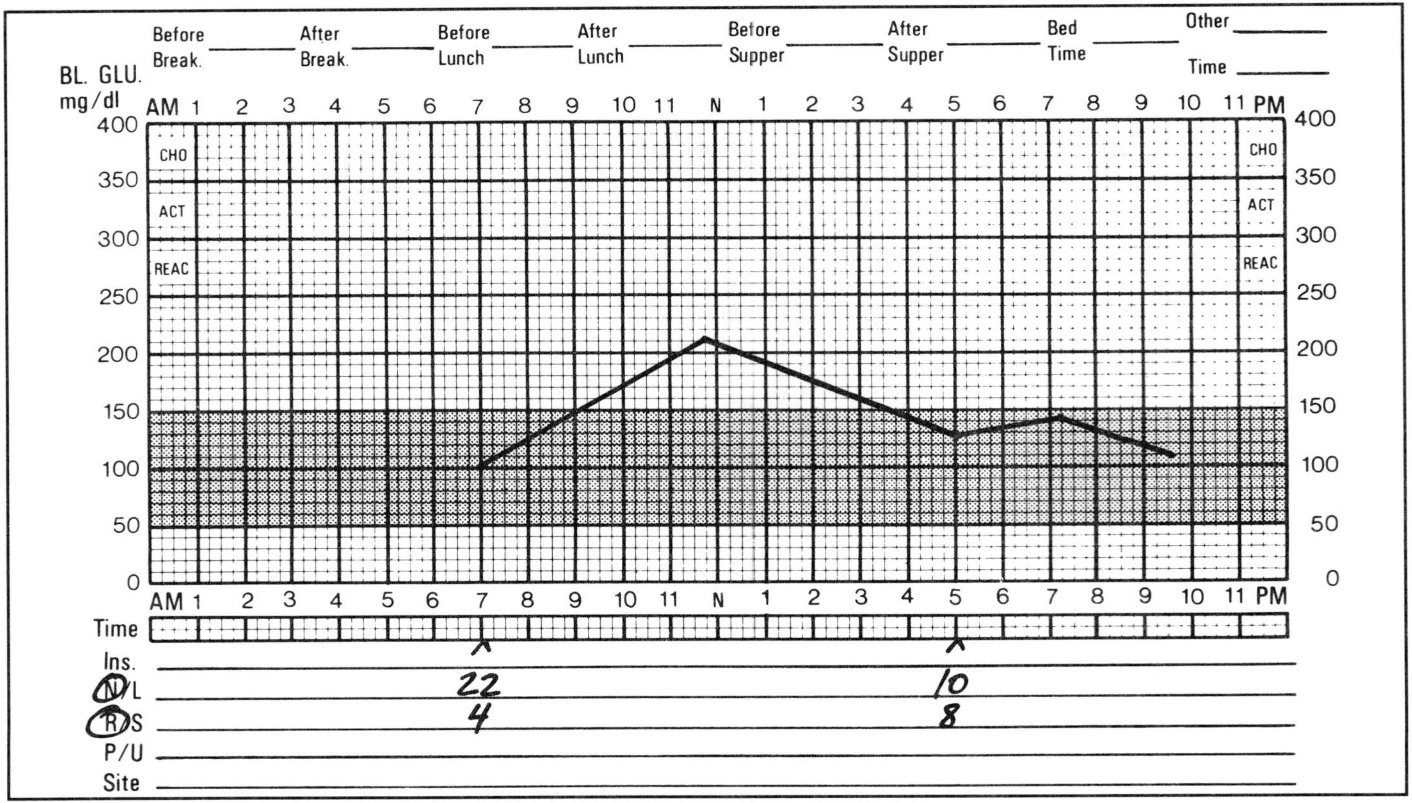

FIGURE 8. Rising blood sugar in the morning.

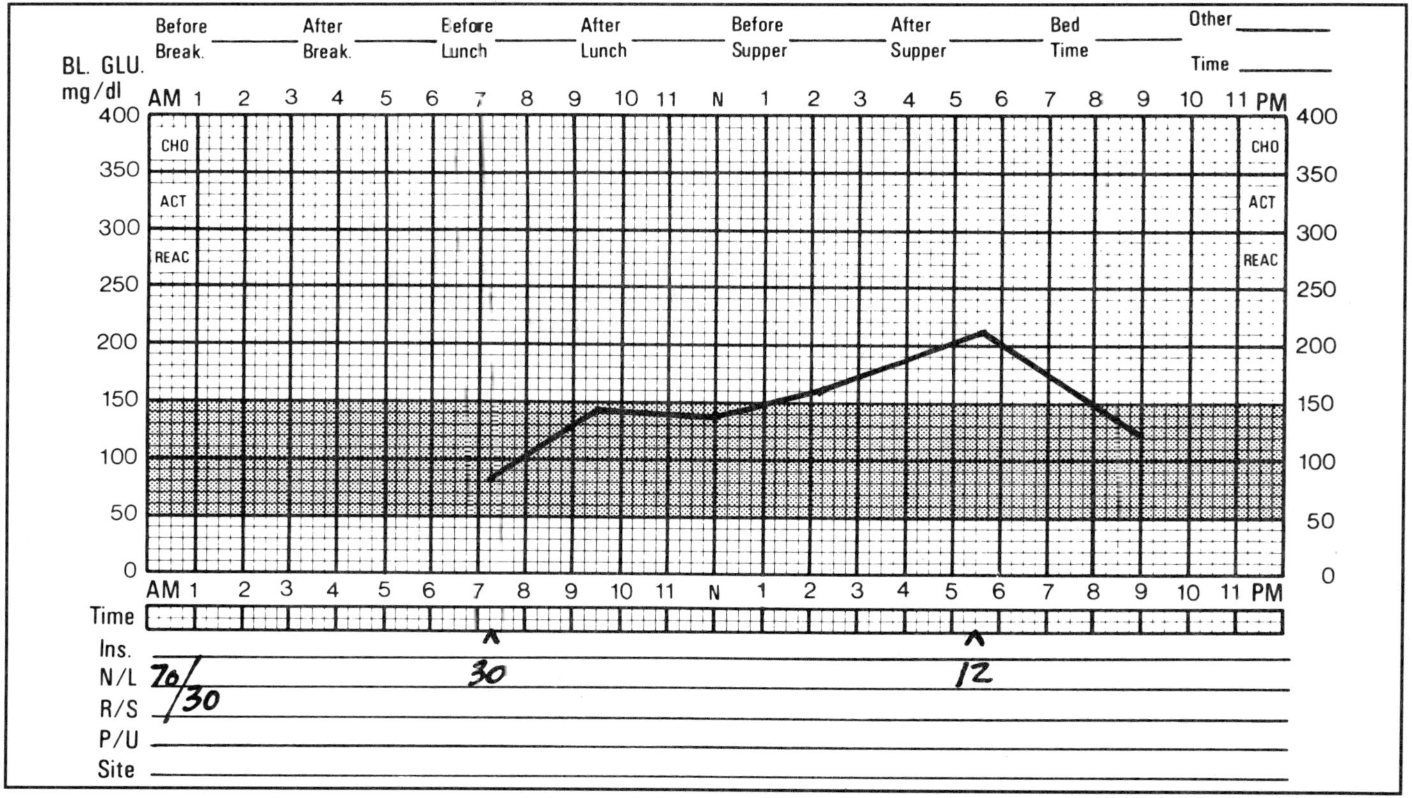

FIGURE 9. Elevated blood sugar levels in the late afternoon.

the 30 units of 70/30 is actually 21 units of NPH and 9 units of Regular). The 70/30 insulin, though ideal for many, was not providing enough NPH to keep afternoon blood sugar normal in this case. The physician suggested keeping the amount of Regular insulin the same since morning glucose levels were fine, but he increased the dosage of NPH. Together with her doctor, this person arrived at a morning dose of 26 units of NPH and 9 units of Regular, which kept blood sugar normal throughout the day.

Figure 10 illustrates rising blood sugar during the evening hours. At first, this person and his doctor felt the best solution would be to increase the amount of Regular insulin he took before supper. However, after further examination of his charts they discovered that he was gradually gaining weight. A close look at his diet revealed that he was consistently eating a larger evening meal than was suggested by his meal plan. Instead of increasing his insulin, he agreed to eat a smaller evening meal. His blood sugar levels returned to normal, and by the next six-month checkup with his physician, his weight had also returned to normal. This is a good reminder that although an easy solution might be to change the insulin dose, it is not always the best solution. *All* aspects of one's chart should be considered before making a change in the management program.

Ups and Downs

Figure 11 (page 26) illustrates the case of a woman who had been testing her blood sugar three or four times daily and felt she was in good control. However, at her last visit to the doctor, her glycated hemoglobin test (HbA_{1C}) was slightly elevated. (A glycated hemoglobin test measures the quality of blood sugar control during the preceding two or three months. A normal level indicates acceptable glucose control over that period. It is a good idea to have this blood test every three to six months to make sure your control is adequate.) The woman was surprised by the high HbA_{1C} result. She had been using the monthly chart but decided to return to daily charting to try to discover the source of the problem. After a week of testing six to seven times per day, she noticed a pattern of rising blood sugar after breakfast. Her level would then return to normal before lunch. Because the glucose level before lunch was normal, she did not change her usual insulin dose. However, since she had been drinking four ounces of orange juice or apple juice with her breakfast, she decided to change her fruit serving to something more slowly digested, such as a small apple or orange. This improved her glucose level somewhat, but her blood sugar level one to two hours after breakfast was still too high. Further examination of her charts revealed that she had been in a hurry in the mornings and was taking her insulin 15 to 20 minutes before breakfast. Her doctor suggested that she take her insulin 45 minutes before breakfast to give the insulin a head start. When she did this, her glucose levels became normal. She decreased her testing to four times daily (before meals and at bedtime), but she also tested one to two hours after meals at least twice weekly to be sure she was in good control.

Figure 12 (page 27) presents a similar problem. This person had high blood sugar levels after breakfast, but his blood sugar level consistently fell too low before lunch. He couldn't detect any problems in his self-management program, so he asked his nurse educator for help. On examination, the nurse educator noticed that only the abdomen was being used for his injections and that some scar tissue had formed. Because he was injecting into the scar tissue, insulin absorption was

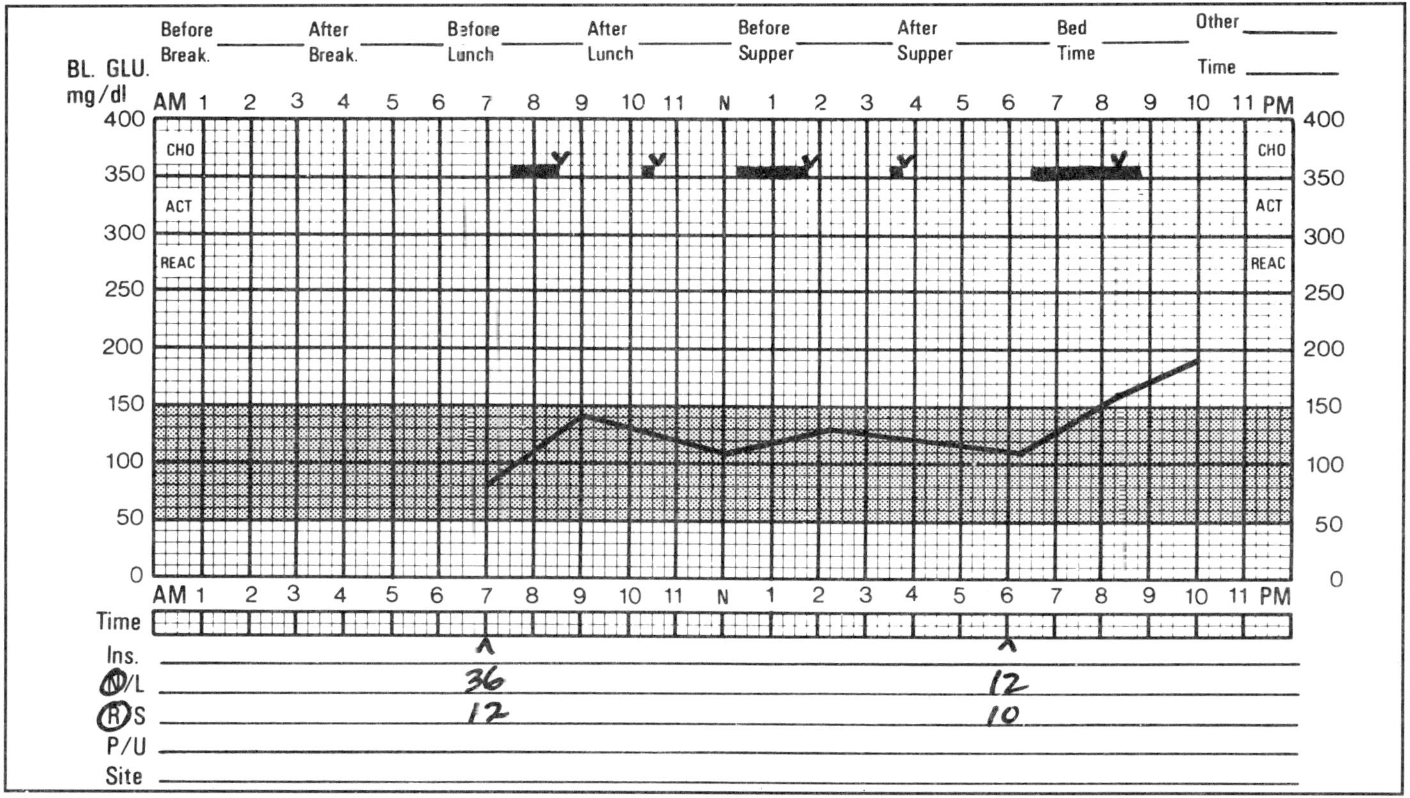

FIGURE 10. Rising blood sugar values during the evening.

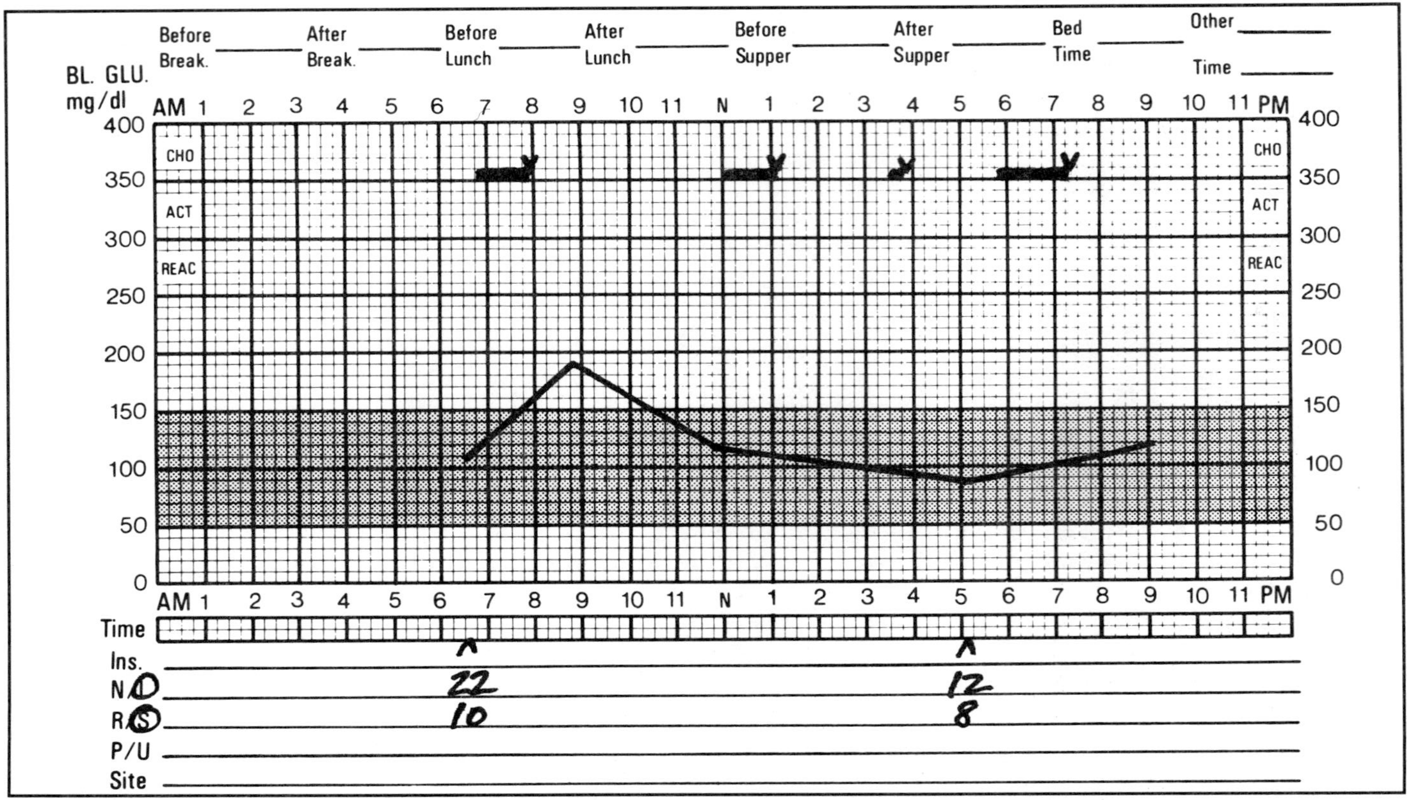

FIGURE 11. Abnormal blood sugar rise after breakfast, with a return to normal levels before lunch.

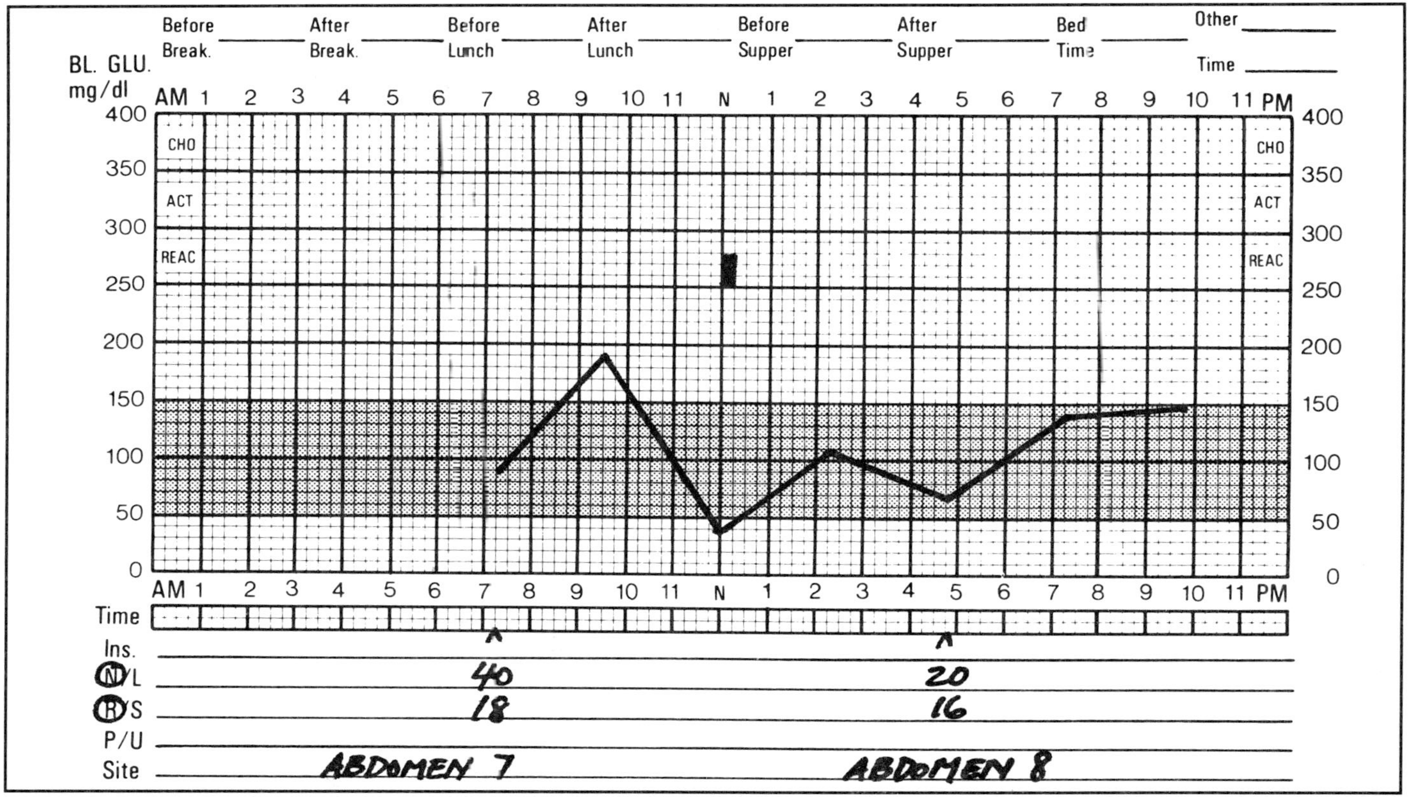

FIGURE 12. High blood sugar levels after breakfast, followed by a plunge to abnormally low levels before lunch.

delayed, resulting in high sugar levels after breakfast. His nurse suggested that he inject into alternative sites on the arms, thighs, and buttocks. With this change, his hyperglycemia after breakfast disappeared, but his blood sugar was still a little low before lunch. He reduced his morning dose of Regular insulin by 3 units and the problem was solved.

The person represented in Figure 13 also noticed high blood sugar levels after breakfast and low blood sugar before lunch. She was in the habit of taking a 45-minute walk at 11:00 AM, about the same time her morning injection of Regular insulin was reaching its peak. She had a flexible schedule, so she decided to take her walk one hour after breakfast instead of at 11:00 AM. This helped resolve the problem, but didn't solve it completely. She consulted her dietitian, and they decided that she should omit her fruit at breakfast, eating it instead as a snack at 10:00 AM after her walk. With these small changes, her blood sugar returned to normal one to two hours after breakfast, as well as before lunch.

Figure 14 (page 31) illustrates a problem that also seems to be related to exercise. This person routinely played tennis three times per week after he left work at 4:30 PM. With the increased exercise on those days, he noticed a pattern of low blood sugar during or immediately following the tennis match. The late afternoon was not the ideal time for him to exercise since his morning dosage of NPH was peaking at that same time. However, his work schedule did not permit him to exercise at another time, so he decided to talk to his doctor about a change in his management program. They discussed two possible solutions for handling the problem: either reduce the dose of NPH on the days when he played tennis, or add a snack to his meal plan before the exercise. Because he did not have a problem with his weight, he chose to eat a snack of one milk, one protein, and one bread exchange before the tennis game. (The snack consisted of one ounce of low-fat mozzarella string cheese, six crackers, and a carton of skim milk.) This snack, which he took shortly before the strenuous exercise, was just what he needed to keep his blood glucose level steady until dinner.

Such factors as stress, hormonal changes, weight loss, medicines containing cortisone or prednisone, and illness, infection, and surgery can all affect blood sugar. Careful monitoring during these times is essential to adjust diabetes medication, if need be, to keep blood glucose levels normal. The next few examples will illustrate the effects these factors can have on diabetes control. Suggested solutions accompany each example.

Effects of Stress

One woman who had been recording her self-management routine on monthly charts recognized two days each month in which her blood sugar was above normal throughout the day. When she examined her chart carefully, she realized that she was under extra stress at work during those particular days. She and her doctor agreed on a slight increase in her morning dose of Semilente and Lente for these days. The problem disappeared the following month. If you find your blood sugar rises after experiencing stress, you might consider other alternatives such as attending a class on stress management or biofeedback techniques. These classes can offer valuable hints to deal effectively with stress so that you can minimize or eliminate the effects altogether and bring your blood sugar back to normal.

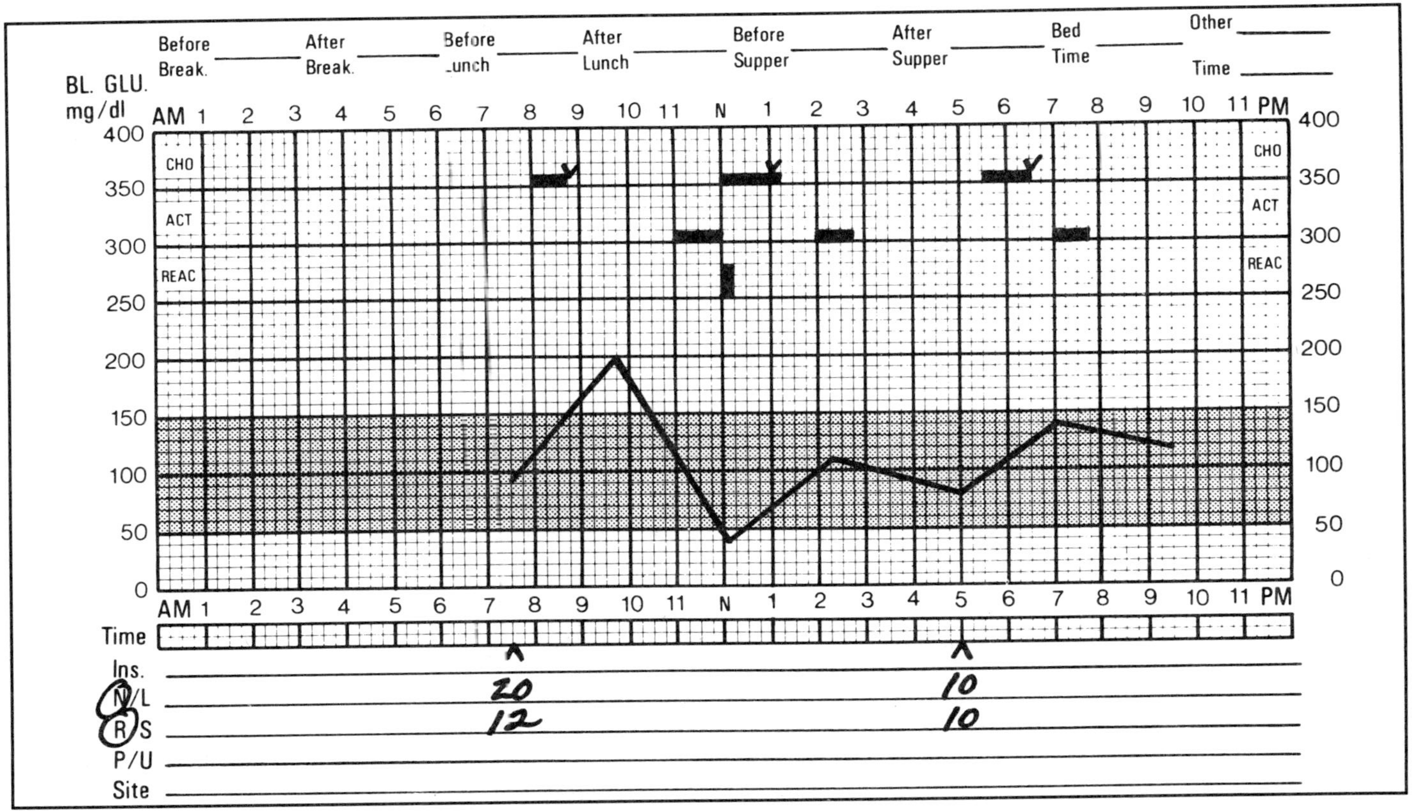

FIGURE 13. A blood glucose pattern similar to Figure 12 but with a different cause and a different solution.

Hormonal Changes

A college student who had achieved relatively good blood sugar control noticed her glucose levels elevated for three to four days before her menstrual period. Since hormones governing the menstrual cycle have a tendency to work against the action of insulin, her doctor prescribed a mild increase in insulin during those particular days each month. Her blood sugar returned to normal as did her glycated hemoglobin test.

Effects of Weight Loss

A 66-year-old man, who was diagnosed with Type II (non-insulin dependent) diabetes nine months earlier, followed a weight-reduction diet, exercised regularly, and took two diabetes pills daily. He tested his blood sugar at various times twice a day and recorded his self-care routine on a monthly chart. He noticed that he felt a little weak and sweaty on several occasions during his midday bowling game. He suspected low blood sugar, and a blood sugar test during these times revealed glucose levels of 50–60 mg/dl. He wasn't sure why he was experiencing low blood sugar, because he followed his diabetes self-management program carefully. He called his nurse educator to discuss the hypoglycemia, and she asked about his weight loss over the previous nine months. After discovering that he had lost 32 pounds, she explained that weight loss and regular exercise had increased his sensitivity to the insulin his body was producing. In addition, his body didn't require as much insulin at his reduced weight. With the doctor's approval, he began to take one diabetes pill per day instead of his usual two. The nurse also explained that when he reduced his weight even further, he might not need to take any diabetes pills at all, a possibility he would need to discuss with his doctor.

Effects of Medication

A woman with Type II diabetes who controlled her blood sugar with diet, exercise, and four diabetes pills per day visited her dermatologist for a severe skin problem. He prescribed a medicine that contained cortisone. However, he first consulted her diabetologist because he knew the cortisone could cause an increase in blood glucose. Since she was taking a large dose of diabetes pills, the doctors decided she needed to switch to insulin before taking the cortisone-containing medicine. After receiving instruction on the use of syringes, insulin, and recognition and treatment of hypoglycemia, she began her insulin and cortisone regimen, checking her blood sugar at least four times daily over the next few weeks. Her insulin was adjusted carefully during this time. After the skin condition cleared and she discontinued the cortisone, the doctor helped her make the transition back to diabetes pills.

No Predictable Pattern

One fellow, after recording his blood glucose for two weeks, found no particular patterns of low or high blood sugar—he simply had many blood sugar readings out of the normal range. After he and his doctor studied his charts carefully, they surmised that some of the swings were due to inconsistent mealtimes and food

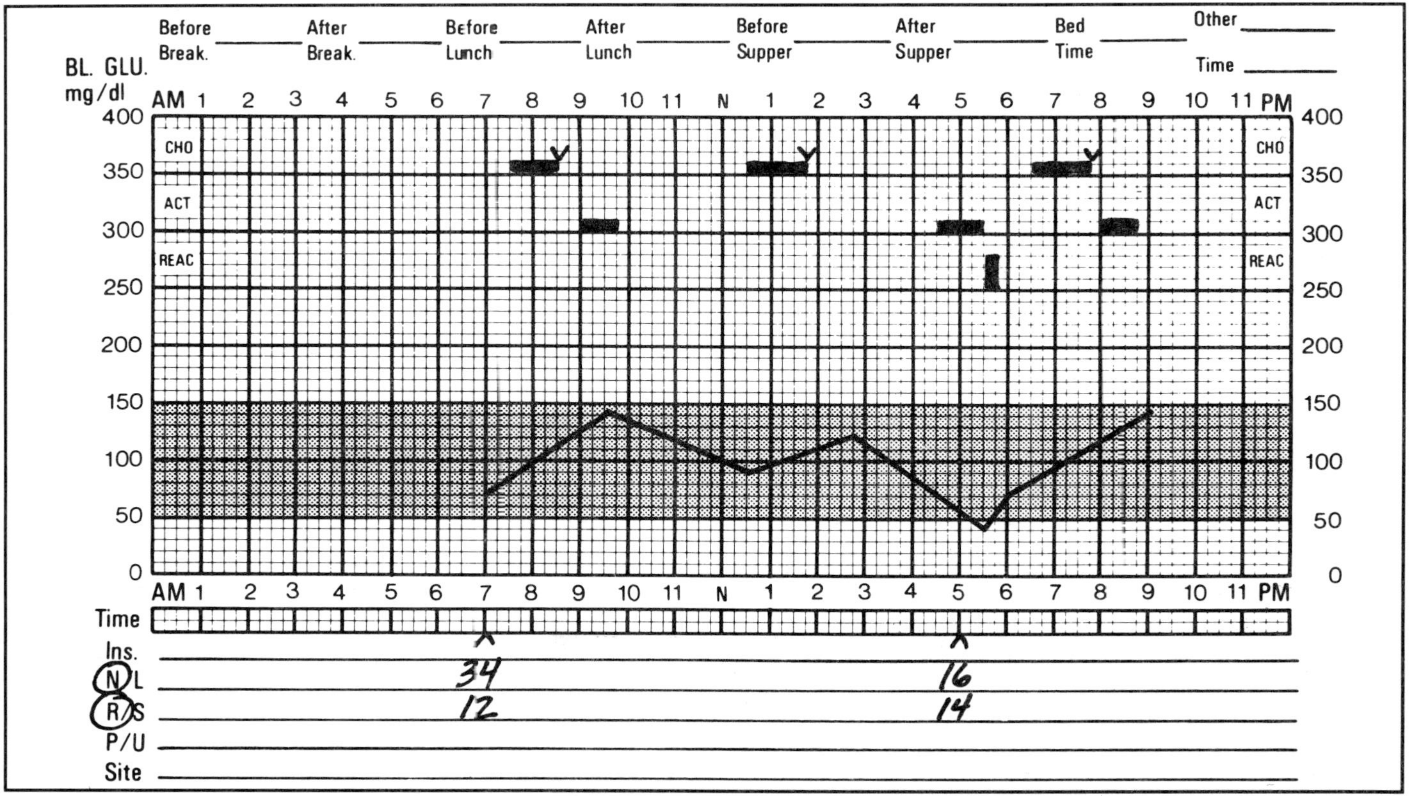

FIGURE 14. A pattern of early evening hypoglycemia that occurred only three times per week (when this fellow played tennis).

amounts from day to day. He agreed to consult his dietitian for suggestions on how to be more consistent with his meal plan in spite of his busy schedule. His doctor also suggested a change in his insulin routine. He had been taking a mix of NPH and Regular before breakfast and before supper. His doctor suggested he take one daily injection of Ultralente and a small injection of Regular before each meal. After a few dosage adjustments during the next few weeks, his blood sugar normalized. An added benefit was the greater mealtime flexibility that his new routine gave him.

PART THREE
CHECKLIST FOR TACKLING CONTROL PROBLEMS

- Don't spend a lot of time trying to figure out why a single blood sugar value is out of line. After recording your glucose values regularly after a few days, try to analyze any *patterns* of abnormal results.
- Make decisions for changes in your management program based on more than just a few tests. Four to seven tests per day for at least a week will be necessary in most cases to make an accurate assessment of the need for change in your program. Of course, more frequent changes may be necessary during times of illness.
- If your blood glucose levels are too high, the best answer is not always to increase your insulin. Though extra insulin may be necessary, remember to evaluate your diet first. It is vital to have a healthy meal plan with a calorie level appropriate to your weight, age, and activity level. Increasing your insulin without bringing your diet under control first can result in unwanted weight gain as well as unpredictable ups and downs in your blood glucose levels. Also, keep in mind that many management problems can be solved by adjusting other components such as timing of activity and injection sites.
- When making changes in your program, it is better to change one aspect at a time to see how it affects your control. If you make several changes at once, you will not be able to determine which has been effective and which has not.
- Don't allow high blood sugar to persist. Many people will dismiss a run of blood sugar values in the 200–300 mg/dl range with the explanation that they will be seeing their doctor shortly and will deal with it then. Each day of high blood sugar could have negative effects on your long-term health, so try to identify and correct problems early. This may require an extra phone call or visit to your doctor.
- Some people settle for poor control with the excuse that their diabetes is simply "brittle." Don't make any decisions until you give a detailed charting system a try for at least two weeks, testing your blood sugar four to seven times daily. Chances are some patterns will become apparent which can be corrected for better control.
- If you detect management problems or your glycated hemoglobin test is elevated, daily rather than monthly charting is valuable for recognizing and correcting problems. If your blood sugar results are stable, you may want to use the less detailed monthly chart.
- Don't wait for your doctor to do all the work. Be your own scientist by discovering your management problems, and work with your doctor to make decisions together which affect your management.
- Give yourself a pat on the back. If you've started testing regularly and recording the different components of your program, you are already charting a course to better control.

Name ______________________ **Day** ____________ **Date** ____________

Weight:	Lbs:	Kg:	Analysis:

Before Break. ______ After Break. ______ Before Lunch ______ After Lunch ______ Before Supper ______ After Supper ______ Bed Time ______ Other ______ Time ______

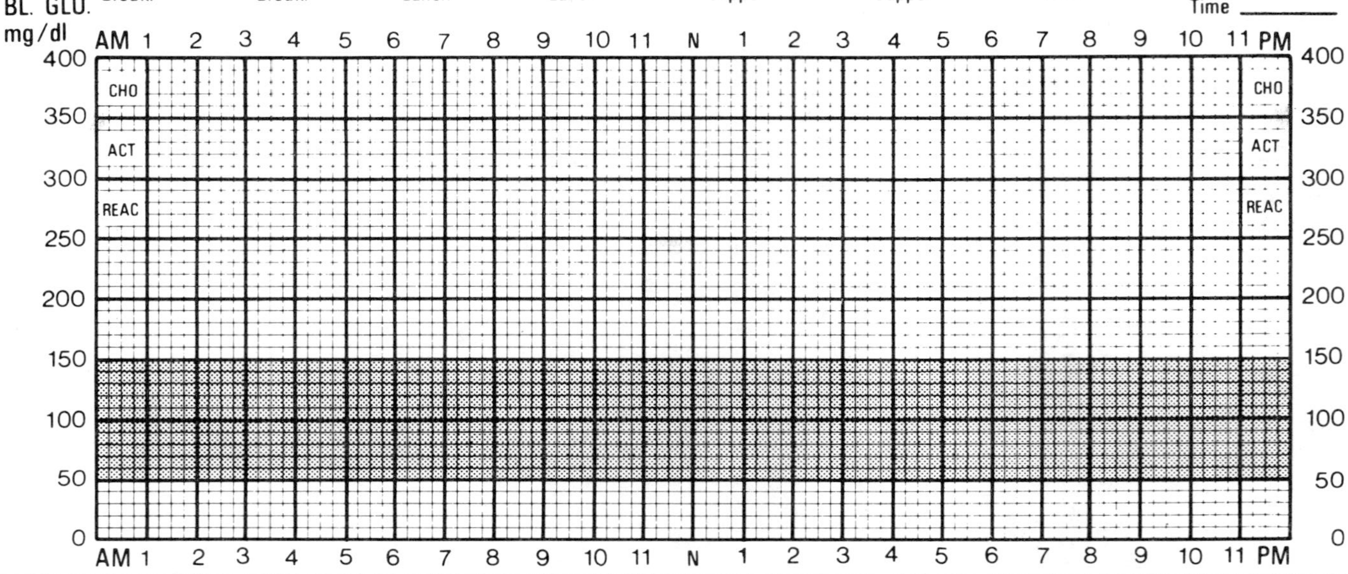

Time	AM 1	2	3	4	5	6	7	8	9	10	11	N	1	2	3	4	5	6	7	8	9	10	11 PM

Ins. ____________________

N/L ____________________

R/S ____________________

P/U ____________________

Site ____________________

BREAKFAST - SNACKS	Quota:		LUNCH - SNACKS	Quota:		SUPPER - SNACKS	Quota:	
Time:	MEA-SURE	GMS CHO	Time:	MEA-SURE	GMS CHO	Time:	MEA-SURE	GMS CHO

Name ______________________ **Day** ____________ **Date** ____________

Weight: Lbs: Kg: Analysis:

Before Break. ______ After Break. ______ Before Lunch ______ After Lunch ______ Before Supper ______ After Supper ______ Bed Time ______ Other ______ Time ______

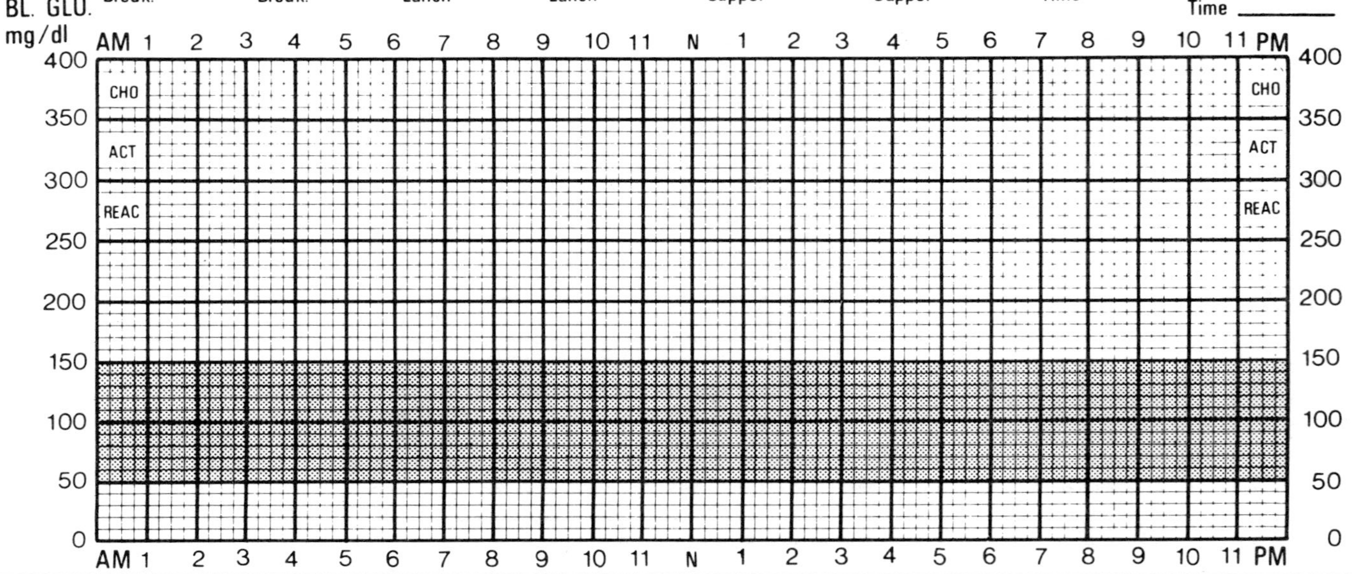

AM 1 2 3 4 5 6 7 8 9 10 11 N 1 2 3 4 5 6 7 8 9 10 11 PM

Time

Ins. ____________________

N/L ____________________

R/S ____________________

P/U ____________________

Site ____________________

BREAKFAST - SNACKS	Quota:		LUNCH - SNACKS	Quota:		SUPPER - SNACKS	Quota:	
Time:	MEA-SURE	GMS CHO	Time:	MEA-SURE	GMS CHO	Time:	MEA-SURE	GMS CHO

WHY NOT GET STARTED NOW?

Get the tools that will give you and your doctor the information you need to make accurate decisions about your self-management. Order a supply of charts today (and an instruction manual) from the nonprofit Diabetes Control Foundation. Find out how great it feels to control your diabetes instead of letting it control you.

Instruction Manual For Blood Glucose Management–
This manual contains complete instructions for using both daily and monthly charts, with examples.

Daily NCR Charts–
Two-part NCR (no carbon required) forms that allow you to keep a copy for your records and to give a copy to your physician.

Daily non-NCR Charts–
Single sheets available in pads of 100 each.

Monthly NCR Charts–
Less detailed than the daily charts, these monthly charts allow you to record four weeks of data on a single form.

PRICE LIST

- Manual only $23.00
- Manual + 50 Daily NCR Charts + 12 Monthlies 30.00
- Manual + 250 Daily NCR Charts 57.50
- 100 Daily NCR Charts 20.00
- 250 Daily NCR Charts 37.50
- Pad of Daily non-NCR Charts 15.00
  (Each pad contains 100 single sheets)
- 12 Monthly NCR Charts 4.50

All prices include shipping and handling. Allow 6–8 weeks for delivery. Send your check (no cash, please) and your order to

Diabetes Control Foundation
Attn: Order Dept.
138-26 58th Avenue
Flushing, NY 11355